Broken Minds

Broken Minds
Saida Chowdhury

ISBN-13: 978-1-912605-83-5

ISBN-10: 1-91-260583-X

This collection published in Great Britain by j-views Publishing, 2025

Text © 2025 Saida Chowdhury

Cover art ©2025 Christiane Sarah Jenkins

All rights reserved. No part of this publication may be reproduced, stored in a retrieval system or transmitted, in any form or by any means, without the prior permission of both the copyright holder and the publisher in writing.

The right of Saida Chowdhury to be identified as the author of this work has been asserted in accordance with the Copyright, Design and Patents Act 1988.

No generative artificial intelligence (AI) was used in the writing of this work. The author and publisher expressly prohibit any entity from using this publication for the purposes of training AI to generate text. Use of AI is intellectual property theft.

j-views Publishing, 26 Lombard St, Lichfield, WS13 6DR

www.j-views.biz

publish@j-views.biz

Contents

Introduction v
Acknowledgements viii
Foreword by Sureena Brackenridge MP. xi
Review by Ian Henery xii
Review by Dr Kuli Kohli xiv
Review by Diyodi Menon. xv
Review by Manjit Sahota xvi
Review by Junna Begum. xvii

1. **Depression & Futility**
   Abyss 2
   A Wall-less Prison 3
   Rambling 4
   Bleak Prospects. 5
   Broken Wings 6
   Our Love Was Never Going To Be Enough 7
   Rambling 8
   Devoid Of Answers. 9
   Help Her? 10
   Inevitable Doom 11
   Invisible Chains. 12
   I Stand In Shame 13
   Maybe 14
   Mental Illness. 15
   Reaching Out 16
   Save Yourself 17
   Shattered 18
   Unspeakable Truths 19
   Unspoken 20
   What Illness?. 21

2. **Love & Strength**
   A Mammoth Promise. 23
   Rambling 24
   Despite 25
   Did I? 26
   Forbidden 27
   Hold Me 28
   I Will Never Judge You 29

Rambling	30
Reality Without You	31
Soar	32
Sum Of Me	33
Use Me As You See Fit	34
Church Poem 15/2/25	35
First Time	36
I Would	37

3. Loathing & Consequence

Rambling	39
Twin Towers	40
Abusive Lover	42
Brainwashed	44
Fuck You (Obsession)	46
Rambling	48
Fury?	49
Ignited Hate	50
Rambling	51
Let Bygones Be Bygones?	52
No More	53
Rambling	54
Nothing To See?	55
Rape Preach?	56
You Let Me Walk Away	58
Genocide In Gaza At Christmas (Again…)	59

4. Searching & Hopeful

Rambling	61
A Billion Stars	62
Can We?	63
Defiance Exhausts Me	64
Don't Suffer In Silence	65
In The Midst Of A Dream (Grenfell x)	66
Keep On Smiling	67
My Refuge	68
I Don't See The Scars	69
Plan Of Action	70
The Worth of Women	71
Rambling	72

About Saida Chowdhury 73

Introduction

This debut collection of poems has been compiled together to bring people face to face with emotions and sometimes, quite troubled emotions at that. The feelings of helplessness, anger, resentment and rage have had a literal outlet through these poems. Sometimes people find that they have no-one to turn to, no-one to listen to their stories without passing judgement and thus these poems are an expression of these repressed emotions, allowing a somewhat peaceful outlet.

From as young as I remember, I always wrote down my feelings, especially when they were wholly negative thoughts. Always being a happy child, when I did try to convey my dissatisfaction about something, I found several things occurred. One, that occasionally my feelings were dismissed as being absurd or as though I had misunderstood situations. And two if I was experiencing melancholic emotions, which occurred later in life, it made people feel sad too. I decided that I didn't want anyone to recreate those sad emotions in someone else or place this emotional pressure or burden on them, so I decided that I would, from then on, write down my emotions and tell The Almighty. Come to think, there were three. The third, being that some people were not emotionally capable of handling such information and I would feel as though, I just let myself down by confiding in someone who was emotionally unavailable, this only served to magnify the feelings of solitude. I soon discovered however, that during the chances where I decided to share my experiences through talking, a great weight had been lifted but the decision to make the changes in my life, ultimately, lay solely in my hands. And no matter how difficult society may have made, making my choices, or I had perceived it to be, the only person who could and still can change things is me.

I was fascinated with the Japanese art practice of *Kintsugi* whereby broken pottery or ceramics are mended using precious metal liquids or lacquer with gold dusting, to highlight the object's cracks or brokenness. This art form promotes the cracks as being an intimate part of the object's history, and having been broken, only makes it more beautiful. The idea is to celebrate the history and the cracks rather than hide them.

I wanted to apply this same philosophy to people, with their physical and emotional scars. Having been broken is nothing to be ashamed about and to remember that the scars are part of you and that they are not something to be hidden but something that is beautiful, to be celebrated and shared. Through sharing we can all learn, help and grow together.

I have constructed this book in four parts: *Depression & Futility, Love & Strength, Loathing & Consequence,* and finally *Searching & Hopeful*.

The reason for doing this is to represent the peaks and troughs of life: even at my lowest points, there would be a sudden smile from a stranger; that embrace that would momentarily take away the pain, or some words serving as a reminder of my worth in this world, when I could no longer see it myself.

I know that this is life for countless people out there. I also wanted to create safe spaces in this book away from potential triggers so that the reader can empower themselves and decide if they want to read about depression or love, as I understand about the emotional consequence of such triggers.

The ramblings in the book are flittering thoughts that came to mind; not entire poems but lines that summed up my outlook at that particular point in time. They have been placed to align with the theme of each chapter.

Regardless of which country you live in, which time period, *Broken Minds* expresses the feelings and experiences that people will experience or know someone to have encountered. This book has taken a journey over twenty years, to show that the feelings are still as relatable today as some of them were back then. Through both first-hand experience and witnessing people's circumstances, I wanted to give a voice to these pains; theses unspoken matters; that burden the minds of so many. For various reasons we decide not to share these burdens, perhaps because of cultural, social or religious restrictions and etiquettes. However, carrying theses burdens can have an immense impact on the mental health and the overall well-being of a person and on a further level, on their social and economic contributions. So being able to share problems and burdens greatly helps people's mental health and society as a whole.

This book chooses to give a voice to those who may not have one or are currently in a position whereby they feel they don't have one. I personally have always found it easier to write down my feelings on paper than vocalise them. There are many people who feel helpless due to their circumstances, situations and societal pressures, and this book not only serves to convey their feelings but also to remind them, that they are not alone, there is always hope and to never, never give up.

I am not and do not claim to be a psychologist or counsellor of any sort. I am merely an observer, fortunate enough to be able to put thoughts and ideas to paper and express them in a way, that is hopefully easily understandable, and relatable.

The purpose of this collection is not to judge but to actually provide a setting, where people aren't judged and can express coherently what they have endured. The book serves as a reminder to people going through their individual challenges in life, that they certainly are not alone and there is help out there.

The book is designed to take the reader by the hand and bring them face to face with situations some people have experienced or are experiencing.

It allows you to come close have a look and leave and then the choice as to what you choose to do with this knowledge is entirely left to the reader.

In a quiet corner or a busy café, read and absorb the words of those "Broken Minds".

Acknowledgements

I am thankful first and foremost to The Almighty for taking me out of the depths of despair time and time again.

As this is my first book to be published, my list of gratitude is long and in no particular order of importance.

Many thanks to Ian Henery of The Ian Henery Show Black Country Xtra part of Black Country Radio, Hugh Ashton of j-views Publishing for so kindly managing all the technicalities of publishing; Christiane Sarah Jenkins Creative Arts & Research Lead at SUIT (Service User Involvement Team) for creating and gifting me the beautiful artwork for the front cover, and Sureena Brackenridge the MP of Wolverhampton North-East for writing and taking the time to write the Foreword. Devinda Diyodi Menon of Creative Connections, Dr Kuli Kohli Wolverhampton Poet Laureate, Manjit Sahota Co-Founder of Poets Against Racism, Junna Begum BADA Strategic Manager & Artistic Director and Legacy WM for their time and incredible reviews.

The team at Legacy West Midlands and Zephaniah Family Legacy Group, Scarlett Ward -Staffordshire Poet Laureate, Tal Singh of Soul Brite Seva, Trevor Latham & Willenhall in Focus, Marion Mansell, Café Royale, Delves Baptist Church Walsall Community, Jeni Sellick - West Midlands House, HBK Solutions Ltd for creating and gifting me my own website, South Asian Women Writers Group, RICNIC, Wolverhampton University, The Heath Bookshop, Poetry Breakfast, Francis of Saturday Books and Claire Birkin from Tales on Tuesday Book Club.

I am so thankful to my Mai, my Abba (who is no longer with us, may he rest in Jannah). Ali, my boys: Taqwan & Ilan and my siblings: Boro Bhaya, Furu Bhaya, Thanni, Rezwan, Sadee, Sandra Bhabi and Tanja Bhabi and their families for putting up with me over the years and giving me that knowledge that no matter what, I will always have a loving, supportive family. Rahida, my sister, a second mum to my boys and the person who has always been a phone call away.

Over twenty years ago, my friend Malcolm told me to publish my poems, seeing them as a survival guide for girls and women. I wish I had the self-confidence and knowledge back then to have fulfilled this. I am so thankful to him for his support and encouragement. My poems and my writing have naturally evolved over time. This baton of encouragement has been taken up by Ian Henery who has been insistent on me in not only pursuing my dream to publish but ensuring it gets completed with the intention to help people, introducing me to some amazing opportunities, experiences and people. He has got 'the cogs' turning again and has also ignited my passion for performing my poetry to an audience.

Years of posting on a social media platform, Missy Margaret has been telling me to publish for years. I have finally done it. I am so thankful for your continual support.

My friends that have always given me incredible support regarding my writing and life. Susan, Nabila, Sunny, Louise & Steve, Sabrina & Richard, Tasha & Sue, Rachel, Jodie, Sarah, Michelle, Janice, Lindsay, Joanne, Madiha, Mobina, Mick, Abi, Sally, The Bradshaw Family, Carmen & Paul, Julie, Katerina, Alan (I wish you could have seen this) and the best next-door neighbours ever, The Johnson family.

Louise – honestly you are just so thoughtful, thank you for always thinking of me and spoiling me.

My new poetry friends, artists & musicians – you are all truly inspirational! Suresh & Dhamiyanthi, Bones, Amy, Sylvia & Andrew Keatley, Lee Benson, Jay Lewis, Francis Sheppard, Glyn Phillips, Cheryl Ann Boot and Katie Victoria thank you for all your advice and chats.

My relatives, for their love, support and interesting debates and discussions which have raised many questions over the years regarding, culture, conventions and conformity.

Anwar Bhai & Bhabi, Limi Mami & Mama, Luton Moi & Mama, cousins & relatives in Brighton, Hillingdon crew def get a shout out!

Shamsuddin Chowdhury always telling me how proud he is and telling me to go for it. Saima Bhabi, Jabin and Hanna Afa, for telling me how important my voice is in discussions about mental health, especially in the Bangladeshi Community.

Khuka Sasa and Sasi, for your encouragement and bringing life and wisdom to every event,

Roma, Shimu Afa, Yagsha, Leena thank you for always keeping it real, you ladies always make me laugh.

Mokhfur Chowdhury, the advice and your support has been invaluable.

Thamim Bhai & Jemeli Bhabi, the calm and sweet addition to every event.

Sazu, Raju and Tipu Bhai for being inspirational with your creativity.

Rafi Ahmed Rahi, always calm and giving such great encouragement and advice.

Rizvi and Shibli Bhai have made me so incredibly happy to hear that I have made you proud.

My sisters-in-law Polly and Shahina, for their love of my poems and continuous support for me, to be me.

The ups and downs of life meant that this book could not have been published at any other time.

I am so thankful to *all* my friends and family, here and abroad and for those who fight for freedom and uphold peace and justice.

I am sorry if I could not mention you all individually, but I do pray for those who have extended their kindness to me and others, to be rewarded abundantly.

To all those people who have in some way, or another helped me on this journey of life, through your ability to make me smile or laugh, your kind words, gestures and actions, you have no idea how much I needed it and for it I am eternally grateful.

Foreword by Sureena Brackenridge MP

Saida Chowdhury may be a new voice in the poetry scene, but she has been quietly crafting her work for over twenty years. Only recently has she found the courage to share her deeply personal and evocative poetry with the world. Her writing, spanning themes of racial discrimination in the post-9/11 era, love, grief, loss, and mental health, is both raw and profound.

This collection is a testament to her resilience – a journey from brokenness to healing, and ultimately, to empowerment. Saida's work is not just about personal catharsis; it is a beacon for others navigating their own struggles. She is deeply committed to the idea of women empowering women and is using her voice to break down barriers, particularly around the stigma of mental health within the Asian community.

I wholeheartedly applaud Saida for her bravery in addressing these issues and for using her poetry as a tool for change. This book is an important and necessary read – one that will resonate, inspire, and encourage healing.

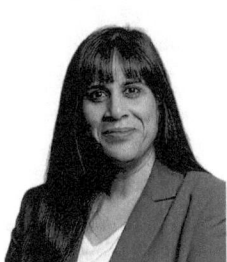

Sureena Brackenridge MP, Wolverhampton North East

House of Commons, Palace of Westminster, London, SW1A 0AA.

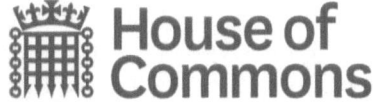

Review by Ian Henery

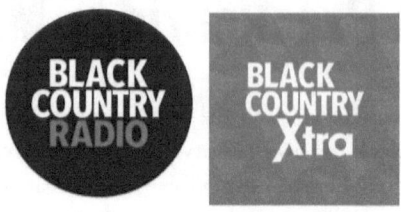

I will never forget the night Birmingham poet Saida Chowdhury walked into a spoken word event called Words of Wisdom at the Café Royale on 27th November 2024 in Wolverhampton.

She had been quietly developing her craft for 20 years and – like a rocket waiting for lift off – she sat behind me, surveyed the room – and booked herself a slot in front of the microphone.

The room went quiet when it was her turn to deliver spoken word, all eyes on Saida – and history was made that night in Wolverhampton.

Saida went on to share her poetry a few weeks later for the Human Rights Celebration Day at the University of Wolverhampton to mark the adoption of the Universal Declaration of Human Rights by the United Nations General Assembly in 1948 – a document that remains foundational to human rights advocacy.

Human Rights and equality is a topic that is very important to Saida who began writing poetry after witnessing the injustices of the aftermath of 9/11 and trying to understand the root causes of abuse that exist in the world.

Her poem, "Genocide In Gaza At Christmas (Again)" was turned into a film by digital creator Diyodi Devinda Menon and screened at the University of Wolverhampton for Human Rights Celebration Day. The film was shared by groups such as Amnesty International, Stop The War Coalition, Save The Children UK, British Red Cross and several Members of Parliament.

And all of this from a poet who had finally found her voice and the empowerment to speak her own authentic truth after walking into a random spoken word event on a dark November evening in Wolverhampton. To be fair, Saida did return to Café Royale for another spoken word event on Winter Solstice 21st December called *All You Need Is Love (and a microphone)* where she performed poems from this book and did a Q&A session with the audience.

Saida was the light that shone in that darkness, the light to illuminate issues that are relevant right now in the world. She burned brightly then and she burns brightly now. She is a star.

Ian Henery
Walsall Poet Laureate 2011 – 2016, 2020 – 2021
Ian Henery Show, Black Country Xtra, Black Country Radio

Review by Dr Kuli Kohli
Broken Minds by Saida Chowdhury

Broken Minds is a collection of poems that offers a poignant exploration of the frustration, anxiety, depression, pain, and irritation arising from the thought processes of young minds in everyday life, reinforcing the reality of mental illness. Personally, I found a deep connection with some of the poems, which resonated with my own early writings where I used to pour my feelings onto paper as a therapeutic exercise—expressing thoughts I believed no one would care about. Saida emphasises this theme throughout her collection.

The book is divided into four parts: *Depression & Futility*, *Love & Strength*, *Loathing & Consequence* and *Searching & Hopeful*. This structure is not only a reflection of the diverse experiences that constitute our mental and emotional landscapes but also serves to highlight the ebb and flow of life. Even at the lowest points, there are moments—a stranger's smile, an embrace—that can briefly alleviate the pain and remind us of our worth, especially when we struggle to see it ourselves. Saida's words are a tribute to the lives of countless individuals navigating these peaks and trenches.

Broken Minds is a good read that sheds light on the complexities of mental health and the resilience of the human spirit. Saida Chowdhury's collection is not just a book of poems but a journey through the struggles and triumphs that define our existence.

Reviewed by Dr Kuli Kohli Honorary Doctor of Letters
Poet Laureate for the City of Wolverhampton 2022-25
Creative Associate for Wolverhampton - Rebecca Swift Foundation
2025-26 www.kulikohli.co.uk

Review by Diyodi Menon

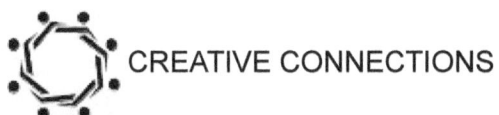 CREATIVE CONNECTIONS

Diyodi Menon
Project Manager | 1in3 Women Empowerment
Project Funded by Arts Council England
Creative Connections itsourright.info

Date: 03/02/2025

To Whom It May Concern,

I first met Saida Chowdhury at the Human Rights Celebration Day on December 10, 2024. Her quiet yet commanding presence filled the room as she read her poetry, touching on topics of resilience, injustice, and healing. That day, her words resonated deeply with me and many others, showcasing the power of poetry to give voice to the silenced and strength to the vulnerable.

Broken Minds reflects Saida's ability to channel raw emotion into poetry that speaks directly to the soul. Divided into four sections: *Depression and Futility*, *Love and Strength*, *Loathing and Consequence*, and *Searching and Hopeful* the collection allows readers to navigate life's challenges and triumphs at their own pace. Saida's use of the Japanese concept of *kintsugi*, celebrating the beauty in scars and imperfections, is particularly inspiring.

Her poem *Genocide in Gaza at Christmas (Again)*, which I had the privilege of adapting into a short film, underscores her commitment to addressing global injustices. Saida's work is more than poetry; it is a call to reflect, heal, and act.

This book is a must-read for anyone who seeks understanding, comfort, or empowerment through the written word. Saida's poetry will leave a lasting impact.

Diyodi Menon – Creative Connections

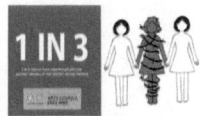 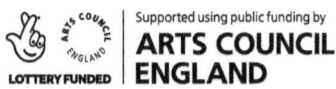

Review by Manjit Sahota
(Co-founder of Poets Against Racism)

Broken Minds is a unique and fascinating collection of poems, a very interesting concept of creating a positive out of something that was once broken.

Saida can write poems that seem both personal and universal at the same time, it's her story but it will connect with so many.

Saida is a powerful, uncompromising poet with a mission to tell her story. This is a great collection, painful, honest, brutal but hits the mark.

The poems leave you with a feeling that through struggle, fightback and resistance, we can grow stronger.

A powerful voice in the poetry world.

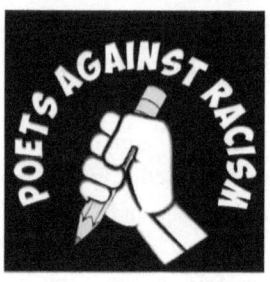

Review by Junna Begum
Artistic Director, Bangla Week

Broken Minds is a powerful anthology of highly original poetry authored by an amazing Bangla heritage poet and activist. Saida brings a deeply moving, unique and refreshing perspective on racial justice, love, grief, loss and mental health. Her poetry achieves the remarkable feat of being simultaneously emotive and contentious, sensitive, passionate and, above all, speaks of a collective truth. Each and every poem is distinctively written, with such precision and clarity, arousing intense emotions. Words of great poignancy span the complexity of our individual existence and the discourse of a nation.

It's difficult to pick a favourite from the collection. For me, *Grenfell* in particular reflects not just the specificity of a singular tragedy but the broader struggles of the marginalised and the final hope offered by love of family. Across the pages, Saida's candid personal journey is laid bare with all its universal resonances. At some point we all experience feelings of anger, frustration and helplessness, but rarely do we voice these feelings. In so courageously sharing the vulnerabilities of her own life, a brave and inspirational champion in the world of poetry encourages each of us to feel and heal – and to recognise that the beauty of these words describes aspects of a journey that is ultimately common to all of us.

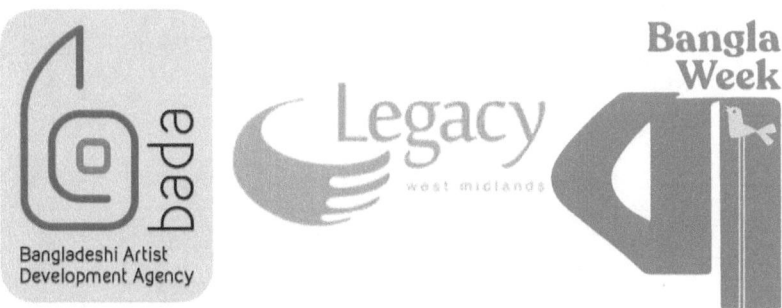

For my parents who named me: the name, meaning happy and blessed in Arabic.

That is all I aspired to be and all that I ever was.

> *In Japan, broken objects are*
> *often repaired with gold.*
> *The flaw is seen as a unique piece of the*
> *object's history, which adds to its beauty.*
> *Consider this,*
> *When you feel broken*

Dedicated to those souls who feel that they are alone in the world.

You are not alone.

Let your voices be heard, for there are those who pray for the silence to be broken.

Broken Minds

by

Saida Chowdhury

j-views Publishing, Lichfield, UK

1. Depression & Futility

Abyss

All this time, I keep on falling,
Into the dark abyss, and it won't help crawling.
Because I'm in too deep and can't get out,
No one can help me, even if I shout.

Unhealthy obsession will bring my downfall,
I pick myself up and then again, I stall.
What is it that I am trying to prove?
Intoxicating, my mind I will lose.

A Wall-less Prison

It's a prison with no walls,
It's a show with no stalls,
I want to say "Fuck You!"
But do I really have the balls?

It's an echo with no call,
It's a bat with no ball,
It's a multitude of impacts,
That reduces a woman to a girl.

It's that tireless motion,
It's the age-old notion,
"Do what duty calls!",
Without a magic potion.

It's a breath holding conquest,
It's an endurance contest,
Sure, it's a battle of wills,
But I'm the one who's suppressed.

It's a reality where everyone's smiles just gleam.
It's a fairytale ending, when the sun starts to beam.
This is what they will have you believe,
Until you see that, which I have seen.

It's futile child, it's a mental disease,
What is this trauma, you are trying to appease?
What are the fragments giving you hope?
These miracles elude you,
Whilst you're smoking your dope.

Bleak Prospects

Something has awoken, that was once asleep.
I'm accustomed to shallow, never venture the deep.

I tried it once, but couldn't catch my breath,
I thought I knew my limits but was out of my depth.

They said they would save me, but forgot to look,
From the realisation, I so fervently shook.

Who can I count on, when my body gets weak?
I'm not quite sure, but my prospects seem bleak.

Broken Wings

My wings are broken, but still, I try to fly,
"The sky's the limit!", but even that's a lie.
In my quest for peace, I battled the storms,
In my pursuit for peace, I took on various forms.

But everyone had their words to say,
I should be living like this, behaving this way.
But I wasn't born, to be subdued,
In my pursuit for freedom, I abandoned my hood.

Live and let live, as long as there is peace,
But when did all the civility cease?
Kip leather hood, designed to make me conform,
But I wasn't born to belong to 'their' type of norm.

A bell at my feet and a distracting transmitter,
Two quite obvious objects as my sole babysitter.
My identity tags, ripped off by my claws,
My feathers are ruffled, but they still hide my flaws.

The skies were mine, I saw the horizons,
But why was it always me compromising?
Nothing lifted me, only weighed me down,
My smile no longer visible, now only a frown.

Now I search for healing, no longer the skies,
My confidence may fool you, but it's all utter lies.

Our Love Was Never Going To Be Enough

Despite my crooked teeth, and crooked nose ....
He loved me.

Despite my dirty mind in a modest world ....
He loved me.

Despite my confessions of guilt ....
He loved me.

Despite snowstorms on a Summers day ....
He loved me.

Despite my visible and invisible imperfections ....
He loved me.

Despite not having a penny to my name ....
He loved me.

Despite being shunned by society ....
He loved me.

He loved me ... for everything that I am,
           for everything that I will be.
But he would 'never' love me...
           for everything that I have been.

Shunned by reality, rejected by life.
This tragedy stands,
on the edge of a knife.

Devoid Of Answers

Why did I tremble with fear, when you were beside me?
Why did I doubt your promise, if you never lied to me?
Why did I shed those tears, if I had no feelings for you?
Why did I get so angry, I still have no clue?

Why am I ridden with guilt, when you brought joy to my life?
Why can't I end this pain, with one slice of the knife?
Why do I still feel, completely devoted, to you?
Why do I know that you still have no clue?

Why do I yearn, for your sole attention?
Why have I given myself a lifetime detention?
Why is this love, so much pain and pleasure?
Why is my love something you cannot measure?

Why doesn't time loop, to give, one chance again?
Why can't I live without having you as a friend?
Why should you have most mercy on me?
Because I beg, from this pain to be finally free.

Help Her?

My mind goes blank,
I try to recall,
Everything that made it go wrong.

Once you laughed, once you cried,
　I tried to help you, but you still had to die.
Little girl, I saw your pain,
　when the sun was shining, for you it was rain.
Nothing could hide the pain you concealed,
　and you went on like it was no big deal.

You painted your face and put on a smile,
　no one can blame you, it was just your style.
You wanted to sell your story to anyone who would listen
　and bring them into your submission.

Wanting to be loved she tried so hard,
　always with strangers, letting down her guard.
What you don't realise is she had so much faith,
　in the goodness of man, but they used it as bait.
As time passed by, she began to think,
　that there's no hope, on a suicide brink.

It wasn't her fault, society let her escape,
　into self-destruction, as she moulded her fate.
So many friends, here and there,
　but only a few that really cared.
Most came along, just for the ride,
　of the excitement and pleasure that she provided.
But no-one really stopped and thought,
　that on their part they were selling her short.

It was all so hard, and all to no use
　and she could no longer put up with the emotional abuse.
If people had just opened their eyes to see,
　we could've stopped all this unnecessary misery.
Now we think, it's better she rests in peace,
　all along putting our minds at ease.
Only "What the hell could we have done?",
　"You could've started by hiding the gun".

Inevitable Doom

Winding stairs, to an inevitable Doom,
She could've stopped it, is what you presume.
But choice wasn't hers, fate led her this way,
This life of self-destruction was here to stay.

Her intelligence and actions were always manipulated,
"It will all be all right!" was what was stipulated.
But she could've stopped it and abolished trust,
But she craved for comfort with an unhealthy lust.
At the bottom of the stairs, she picks herself up,

Realistic, optimist, never gives up.
She stumbles to her feet again,
Doomed to repeat again,
Mistakes and promises that's she's going to break again,
Until it comes to the point, that she just won't wake up again.

Invisible Chains

Invisible chains… impossible task …
"Is everything OK?" is all they seem to ask.
A sugar-coated version is what I tend to give,
'Cos they can't possibly fathom how I really live.
My soul so delicate, and wholly raw,
With every confession, revealing my core.
An enigma, spectacular, under lock and key.
But perhaps if I shared, I could finally be free.

I Stand In Shame

I stand in shame, I want my slate wiped clean,
There are places I wish that I had just never been.
There are places which, I wish, I didn't know exist,
But at the time, Satan called, I just couldn't resist.

I stand in shame, I want my book erased,
With a pure beginning could it really be replaced?
With pure intentions, could it please be rewritten?
But why did I choose all those things that were so clearly forbidden?

I stand in shame; I want my song withdrawn.
And though the melody plays, I sense a new dawn.
And though the melody adapts, there is a chance for change,
All now perceivable in my optimistic range.

I stand in shame, I took a life to save mine,
And though history is hidden, I still do the time.
And though history adapts to realign truth,
I'm alone confessing sins in my solitary booth.

Maybe

Maybe I don't go out at night, because I know what darkness hides.
Maybe they had convinced me it's safe, but now I know they lied.

Maybe I've seen darkness, that overpowers the light.
Maybe I've seen demons, that make you wish you forego sight.

Maybe I have seen fear, like you can't even fathom.
Maybe I've seen despair, beyond what you can imagine.

Maybe I've seen power, being unjustly used.
Maybe I've been helpless, to aid the abused.

Maybe I've heard voices, that were deliberately muffled.
Maybe I was the one, who had their plans ruffled.

Maybe I was cursed, to see all this horror.
Maybe I was blessed, to acknowledge 'their' sorrow.

Maybe it's my duty, to reveal what I've seen.
Maybe I could, if only my lips could now speak.

Mental Illness

It became an illness, that I had fought.
I thought it was an illness, that time had lost.

All swept under my magic rug,
But this was a feeling, that I just couldn't shrug.

Why did it resurface, out of the blue?
I wish I knew why, but I haven't a clue.

Why did it encroach on my daily life?
Every day is an effort, my constant strife.

Reaching Out

I spend my nights, awake and thinking,
Into this bottomless pit, I'm continuously sinking.
And though I reach out, nothing tangible avails me,
All my screams and shouts, even my voice now fails me.

How did I come to stand so close to the edge?
I attributed wings, to your beautiful pledge.
I waited so eager, for this promise of rescue,
It wasn't contrived, just as a means to test you.

How far do I have to fall, before you come?
The deeper I fall, I lose sight of the sun.
I'm still reaching out, but it's getting scarily darker,
And now my reality becomes undeniably starker.

Save Yourself

Save yourself, from the madness that I project,
Save yourself, from something that I can't protect.
Save yourself, it a question of time,
Before the fragments disperse and I lose my mind.

Save yourself, you know I can swim,
And this final time, I won't let you dive in.
Save yourself, I've gained so much strength,
And despite the injury, I can do the length.

Save yourself, I won't drown in the flood,
Save yourself, I'm not worth spilling your blood.
Save yourself, I can see the shore,
I don't think your mind can take much more.

Save yourself, this battle is personal,
We've seen it many times, we've had the rehearsal.
Save yourself, you know the means of escape,
But you still contemplate on how we relate.

Save yourself, I know where the life ring resides,
You still have time, before you're swept away with the tides.
Save yourself, it's your last chance to be free,
Save yourself, before you're engulfed by the sea.

Shattered

Shattered ...there seems to be a billion fragments,
The once pure water, now lies there stagnant.

No point in getting on your knees, to pick them up,
No point in trying to fill this once full cup.

Shackled by convention, what is this indeed?
Can you not see that I have an emotional need?

Shattered are my dreams into tiny fragments,
So still is this water, that's now become stagnant.

Unspeakable Truths

Why do my lips have to reveal unspeakable truths?
Why do I have to feel pain, to provide them with proof?
From the corners of my mind, I try to comprehend my trauma,
They say, I'm attention seeking, manifesting my own drama!

Little do they know, my voice had been silenced,
I endured for too long, this emotional violence.
But I saw the sun rays as a symbol for hope,
Reality had a become a pill, designed only to choke.

Nothing was sugar coated, true and bitter,
I couldn't erase this anguish, by just getting fitter.
I have stories to tell, of unspeakable truths,
But only my tears to provide them with discernible proof.

Unspoken

I fear for my mind and the burdens it bears,
I fear for my life, but who fucking cares?

I'm sullen, I'm lonely, there's people around me,
I can't look back; there's demons behind me.
They chase me, they haunt me, they live in desire,
They want to lead me to the perpetual fire.

There's routes, there's avenues, there's means of escaping,
But this painted smile hides my soul that is breaking.
There's laughter, there's joy, but there's also shame,
I pray that they never remember my name.

What Illness?

I suffer from an illness, that leaves me weak,
That makes all my prospects, seem bitterly bleak.

I suffer from an illness, whose secrets I hide,
And the illness it worsens, the more I keep it inside.

I suffer from an illness, that imprisons my soul,
And all the over-thinking, takes a devastating toll.

I suffer from an illness, that removes my esteem,
That erases my smile and dullens my gleam.

I suffer from an illness, from which I have to pretend,
And on prescribed medication, they try to make me depend.

I suffer from an illness, that has no cure,
And though my actions are erratic, my heart is pure.

I suffer from an illness, which is no way clear,
And from potential triggers, I must always steer.

I suffer from an illness, some try to refute,
But there's no point partaking, in a ridiculous dispute.

I know my illness, as it slowly claims me.
The invisible destroyer, that they just can't see.

2. Love & Strength

A Mammoth Promise

You made that promise, so where are you now?
"You'll never be alone" was your solemn vow.
You'd wrap me up in cotton, and cover my ears,
You'd be my only supporter, in a crowd full of jeers.

The promise was mammoth, but so was your love,
A special blessing for me, sent from above.
It's a piece of mind, that can't be bought.
It's the reaffirmed healing, that I earnestly sought.

Your love knows no time frame, it's ageless to me,
But it's locked in our minds, clandestinely.

In your mind I'm ageless, In your mind,
I'm carefree.
In your mind I'll be,
Whatever you want me to be.

Despite

Despite my crooked teeth, and crooked nose ....
He loved me.

Despite my dirty mind in a modest world ....
He loved me.

Despite my confessions of guilt ....
He loved me.

Despite snowstorms on a Summers day ....
He loved me.

Despite my visible and invisible imperfections ....
He loved me.

Despite not having a penny to my name ....
He loved me.

Despite being shunned by society ....
He loved me.

He loved me... for everything that I have been,
                for everything that I will be,
                for everything that I am.

Did I?

Did I mesmerise you, with the words that I said?
Did I mesmerise you, when I turned my head?

Did I steal your heart, from its locked cage?
Did I steal your sadness, and leave you dazed?

Did I lift your moods, to skies unseen?
Did I lift you to places, that you've never been?

Did I erase your tears, with a gentle stroke?
Did I erase your fears, and enlighten hope?

Did I steady your hands, when they started to shake?
Did I steady your heartbeat, every time it did break?

Did I carry your laughter, over mountains so high?
Did I carry your burdens, that made you cry?

Did I embrace the passion, from words untold?
Did I embrace the truth, from the dice that were rolled?

All these moments, capture the essence of me?
Which will stay in your mind, for an eternity.

Forbidden

It's forbidden for me ... to call out your name,
It's forbidden for me ... to say, "I feel the same".
I have to commit to the path that I have chosen,
But from the depths of my soul, these emotions have 'rosen.

It's forbidden for me ... to give you that look,
It's forbidden for me ... to open my book.
And though the pages yearn to be turned,
But from stories long told, there's lessons I've learned.

It's forbidden for me ... to touch your face,
It's forbidden for me ... to long for your embrace.
And though you're clearly there, I must resist,
But these feelings are mutual and still persist.

It's forbidden for me ... to feel your breath on my skin,
That's far too close, I mustn't give in.
But as our eyes meet, there's mutual respect,
This secret love, we shall forever protect.

Hold Me

Hold me in madness, hold me in fear.
Hold me in darkness, so that I know that you're near.

Hold me in moonlight, hold me in day.
Hold me so tightly, that my fears fade away.

Hold me in war, hold me in peace.
Hold me until, my tears come to cease.

Hold me in joy, hold me in pain.
Hold me so I know that I am still sane.

Hold me when the sun, blisters our skin.
Hold me when the ice, freezes us from within.

Hold me when I'm trembling and steady my hand.
Hold me when there's no more, grains of sand.

Hold me when the silence, deafens our ears.
Hold me, from now, till the end of our years.

Hold me through fights, when words aren't enough.
Hold me for forever, if I'm who you love.

I Will Never Judge You

I invested all my strength to tell you the truth.
Don't really know what I was trying to prove.
Don't really know what I expected you to do.
But as soon as I did, you came clearly through.

A blessing is statement, "I will never judge you".

Piece by piece, you lightened my load.
Your generosity had my head about to explode.
The joy contracted, nearly had me implode.
Because only you knew what you had to decode.

I carried a burden which was getting too heavy for me.
But it was something that society didn't want to see.

This feeling is something completely
unrivalled.
I look to you,
for my mental survival.

Reality Without You

I stand with arms wide open, ready only for your embrace,
A reality without you, is something I just can't face.
This silence is deafening, but so are my cries,
The longer you're absent, the more of me dies.

I convince myself, that it's for the best,
You don't have to hear everything, that I have to confess.
Your reality continues, in an alternate world,
Where I'm reduced to nothing, but a faceless girl.

Bade your farewell, and live out your dreams,
I don't want you to witness, how I fray at the seams.
I don't want you to be the one, to observe my demise,
How much I really love you, will leave you so surprised.

Soar

We could talk for hours, without taking a breath,
Despite your intellect, I never felt out of my depth.
That was how you nurtured my essence, and lightened up my soul,
Every word you uttered was tinged with gold.

This is a solo mission, Gorgeous, so off you fly,
I never thought that I would be able to say, "Goodbye".
But this time, that's it, I think we have reached our limit,
Now it's time for you to take on the summit.

Don't let the weights of the past weigh you down,
Because from the memories, we have monumentally grown.
Stronger now, we know who we are,
Don't let my memory be an emotional scar.

With every breath, you will certainly heal,
With my every confidence, again you will feel.
You deserve the stars, to mirror your shine,
She will cross your path; it's a question of time.

Sum Of Me

I'm a plethora of emotions, simultaneously abounding.
I'm a sum of all my fears, miraculously compounding.

I'm a multitude of sins, in an innocent form.
I'm a misfit with a face, trying to fit in the norm.

I'm a recognised race, with a place in society.
I'm a symbol who must, assume simple propriety.

I'm an emotional wreck, who must smile, to save face.
I'm a little busy body, all over the place.

I'm a deserted soul, left to wander the world.
I encompass everything I am, from a woman to girl.

Use Me As You See Fit

If I was a pencil, would you sharpen my point?
If I was a compass, would you strengthen my joint?

If I was a ruler, would you straighten my line?
If I was a sandglass, would you let me run out of time?

If I was a highlighter, would you let me stand out bold?
If I was a thermometer, would you let me show you cold?

If I was the case holding everything in?
Would you let me tear at the seams and spill at the brim?

If I were colours, would you let me brighten your picture?
If I was a pencil, would you mask my conjecture?

If I was a rubber, would you let me erase your mistakes?
I will be whatever you wish, if that's what it takes.

Church Poem 15/2/25

(Delves Baptist Church – Walsall)

We live in peace and choose to pray,
Even if storm Darragh blows the rooftop away!

We won't let a missing roof, stop us from praying,
We stand firm in our faith, and this is where we're staying!

How beautiful it is, for a community to come together,
Through joy and sorrow and despite the weather.

But this is the beauty that enlightens hope,
Through God and prayer is our way to cope.

That nothing no wind, no roof, will make our faith falter,
For we will continue to pray even if all that remains is this ancient altar.

First Time
14/1/25

The first time in decades that I no longer fear the weather.
I no longer meticulously look it up, looking at what each hour may bring.

I no longer fear the rain, the wind, the frost…
For I had lost myself to worry at an exponential cost.

What happened? I hear you ask.
The first time that you said you saw me … the real me …
It was the first time that the veil had ever been lifted.
It was the first time that I saw myself as whole.
It was the first time that the pernicious weight had been removed from my shoulders.
It was the first time that perfection was something that I no longer sought…
As that was how you viewed me through your eyes.

The first time in decades that I no longer fear the weather.
The first time that true love, as pure as its intentions, warms me.
The first time that true love, shelters me.
The first time that true love, protects me from all of life's elements.

I have waited a lifetime … for this 'first time'.

I Would

I'll catch those stars when they crash and burn,
I'll take your punishment, when it comes to your turn.
I'll can't heal your wounds, although I can try,
I promise, I'll never make you cry.

I'll give you that promise, for which you've been waiting,
I'll abolish those demons, that your mind keeps creating.
I'll blunt those knives, so they can't harm you,
I'll give you that apology, you're so overly due.

I'll hold my breath, for you to catch yours,
I'll make every opportunity, open your doors.
I'll limit the barriers, between you and success,
I'll never make you feel, like you're worthy of less.

I'll manifest your dreams, to make you believe,
I'll draw all of things, which you can achieve.
I can be that step, if you just can't reach,
I promise I'll listen, and not just preach.

I'll tell the truth, for it's been a long time standing,
I'll write letters, protest, but now I'm demanding.
I can't bring children to light, for the world that we're in,
For we're not just expanding but imploding within.

I'll hold them back, whilst you make your escape,
I'll make sure there's no outline, for official tape.
I won't stand in silence, when justice is due,
But you would do this for me, as I would for you.

3. Loathing & Consequence

*Why did you teach me to speak,
If I'm not allowed a voice?
Why did you teach me about freedom,
And then give me no choice?*

Twin Towers

The attack on Twin Towers was a struggle of powers, between west and east and humanity ceased.
As Blair put it in his polemical case, the whole masquerade was just a disgrace...
On the civilised world of values and peace and finally give commemorance to the deceased.
Listen people, I know it's the past, but the repercussions will inevitably last,
Where westerners must be paranoid to survive, 'cos if Al'Qaeda find you, you won't be alive.
I'm sad to hear that so many died, and in my sadness I even cried.
One thing that we can't neglect, as I ponder carefully and reflect.
One small group did it to a nation, so Bush tears up Afghan with his invasion.
What did the women, children and elderly do? That they had to put up with this tyrannical abuse?
As they fled their homes and went to Pakistan,
And suffered for nothing at the cause of Bush's plans...
To wipe out terror or was it revenge? No matter what, it won't make amends.
Each country has its own little terror, with the IDF, IRA and even ETA.
But who intervened when it was between two small lands?
Instead, distributed weapons right into their hands ... to almost fuel a violent storm.
Sounds like terror? But it's the norm.
Then a superpower gets attacked, and now the people have to watch their backs...
For terror that already rules the world, and media goes on to specifically mould...
Our judgement into bias thinking, almost the same as alcohol drinking.
Irrational, hasty, clouded conclusions, that lead to nothing but mass confusion.
So many don't know what side of the fence, that they should stand on, in their line of defence.

Whilst others go on to blindly ignore, what surrounds them seems to be an eyesore.
The treatment of others they choose to neglect, and in them an ignorance I detect.
They want no pain and want no sorrow, but if you don't help others, it'll be you tomorrow.

Abusive Lover

We know … a destructive combination, no good for each other,
But is solitude better than my abusive lover?
All the things he said, goes around in my head,
It's too much for me, I'm better off dead.

The words of the abused are so heartfelt,
To encounter such emotions, makes one melt.
Whilst the abuser continues his destruction again,
Feeding insecurity is the aim of his game.
He thrives on knowing that he has so much power,
So that in the fear of his presence, you tend to cower.

See somewhere in his life, he learnt it was right,
To freely do anything he wanted, day or night.
The insecurity though, is embedded in him,
Lost sight of religion, so nothing is a sin.
Morals and values have been disposed,
But he said he loved you, when he first proposed.
See, slowly, slowly you discover his act,
But you can't leave him now, 'cos you made a pact.
It's so sad that so many have to depend,
On these violent, cruel, unloving men.
A slap in the face, and it's always, "I'm Sorry!"
"I'll never do it again!" same old story.

You know and I know that you've heard it all before,
But it's always a struggle getting to that door.
You're lucky that you have got him, is what he says,
But behind your back, indulging in affairs.
This ego, this malice, must be defeated,
Because in all of his promises, it's you that he's cheated.

You were better without him, and you will much better after,
And we will finally hear the sound, of the once silenced laughter.
Freeing yourself, is your objective,
Finding the right man, means being selective.
I know it's easier said than done,
But whilst you're with him, you're nothing to none…
That is of course only in his eyes,
Why don't you get up and leave and give him a surprise.

That you don't need anyone to give you abuse,
When you walk out the door, tell him "You lose!".
Then he'll want you back, because he's seen that you're strong,
And that with him is "where you always belong".
Cut the bullshit, cut the crap,
You can see from this shit; it's a fucking trap.
But you're not with the mice, you're with the men,
So, say to his face, "fucking come again?"

"You had your chance and you fucking failed,
I discovered your plot, and had you nailed.
When you learn to treat others with more respect,
You will no longer be a man that I detest.

Brainwashed

Your sweet caress was what I longed for,
But these days it doesn't matter anymore.
Unrequited love is always bitter,
And now I realise, I will let it from me flitter.

I know now that I'm better than that,
You bitching at me even calling me "fat".
I was brainwashed to think that you cared for me,
But now reminiscing has shaken that tree.

'Till late late hours I would wait for your call,
And then into the same trap, I would fall.
Longing, made me want to hear your voice,
And although I tried, I had no choice.

I dialled your number and rang you again,
Almost making me feel sub-human.
What's the trick, I dialled, and I dialled,
And always fell, for that fucking smile.

It was true, I was fooling myself,
Thinking that I didn't need anybody else.
But your actions showed you up, you fucker!
"Don't touch me, I'm not your lover!"

Saying "no" is going to be hard,
But now I know who's dealing the cards.
The more I listen the more I ignore,
The more you play, the higher I score.

It gets me vexed when you say, you knew I would call,
Wait a minute boy, get ready for a fall.
So many flies get attracted to honey,
I don't want you; I just want my money.

As clear as crystal, I'm through with you,
What are you going to say, what are you going to do?
Nothing, because this time I'm much stronger,
And I can't put up with this bullshit any longer.

Being with you was an irrational choice,
You never let me have an opinion or even a voice.

Just because you shout, doesn't mean you're a man,
And then using violence, doesn't prove it again.
I try to stay calm and maintain my composure,
But I can already see that my intelligence has lost ya!

Fuck You (Obsession)

Fuck you and your fucking thoughts,
A mistake has been made, and this is what it's taught,
Not to give it all up, and receive a pile of shit,
I'm not so emotional, I'm a realistic bitch.

Because you're stressing me out, with your paranoid fits,
I'm only flashing my cleavage, because I love my tits.
You say I'm so damn perfect, but it's only for you,
But you're clamping me down, and you know it's all true.

I just want to be myself, who I really am,
Confidence doesn't mean, that I want another man.
But it definitely shows you up, and your true colour,
You're not leading an example, that other men should follow.

I can't be fucked, with all this obsessive crap,
You say you want me to yourself, but it's just a trap…
Strap …with this gun to my waist,
I point it at you and react in haste ….
Sweat …dripping down my spine,
I jump out of bed and realise everything's fine.

Dreams express, my repressed emotion,
Bottle it up, because it will cause commotion,
Like an irritable rash, all over my skin,
Don't confuse the elements, of Yang with the Yin.
I can be harsh as a bitch, or sweet as pie,
I can tell you the truth, or just blatantly lie.
But all this is dependent on your disposition,
I follow on closely, don't doubt my precision.
If you're honest to me, I'm honest to you,
Want me to cry? Then fucking boo hoo!
Want me hurt? Want me in pain?
You can't defeat me, because I mastered the game.

I will always be on a level above,
Because the pain you caused, definitely isn't love.
You can leave me so easy, and then show that you're in pain,
The way you act, is just so fucking lame.
So please for once, just grow up,
'Cos else you'll get stuck at the bottom, and lose sight of the top.

So much pain, and so much pleasure,
Taken for granted, at your leisure.
But you won't excel, you will only fall,
'Cos you stopped my tracks, so now fucking stall.

*This smile is pretty, but it is painted,
My heart was pure, but now it's tainted.*

Fury?

I can't decide, is it fury or is it rage?
But I should unleash this power from its destructive cage.
I'm left in awe, are you in denial?
Through your own words, you're putting yourself on trial.
Sweet speech was one, you thought you had mastered,
But you chat that shit, when you're completely plastered.
What's the difference? You'll never change,
And when I refuse, it is me that is strange?
See your style's the same, from when we were together,
Just 'cos you're preaching, it doesn't mean that you're better.
Hypocrisy lies not only in your eyes, but also your soul,
To deceive me, I can see, is your only goal.
I don't understand what you're trying to establish?
Are you trying to win me, or my esteem extinguish?

Ignited Hate

Ignited hate, created by your disposition,
Fuelled my anger, but yet you held your position.
Admit you're wrong and prove your manhood,
But by your words, you firmly stood.
So revenge is best, when it's served cold,
And your little story I did unfold.

I'm trapped in this maze of my mental feud,
My actions are classed as irrational, some may think they are rude.

Ignited fire, leaves me turning,
In my never-ending hatred, you'll always be burning.
Let the flames surround you and scorch your skin,
Looking for an exit, you start to spin.
There's no escape now, you have to pay your debts,
On the first day we met, you claimed, "let's … "
"Become a couple, eventually get married",
With all your promises, my hopes you carried.
Then one fine day, it came shattering down,
You didn't mean to make me look like a ridiculous clown.
But I took off my paint, and wanted revenge,
See it's my respect and honour, that I had to defend.
So, stay where you are, and burn in your flames,
I've no time to listen to your apologetic claims.

Is there an escape from this invisible hold?
I tried to fit the unfit-able mould.
It's not that bad is easy to say,
but is it enough to make me stay?

Let Bygones Be Bygones?

They ravaged my body, but never took my soul,
To satisfy their lust, was their only goal.
But no apology, "Let Bygones be Bygones!",
But you should've asked me, as the one who's been wronged.

Don't take me for a fool, because I choose to be silent,
I don't want to pave the way, for people to be violent.
But between me and them, only God is our witness.
But I assume you forgot, when you happened to pursue this.

This barbaric act, of deplorable shame,
It sickens me to my stomach; I can't even remember your names.
But that's what you desired, unaccountable deeds,
And I pray for your punishment on my worn-out beads.

No, I'm no saint, you put me up there,
If you burnt in hell, I really wouldn't care.
Because you knew the lines but still exceeded your step.
Your integrity is something that you should've kept.

But behind closed doors, the evil won,
You did what you did, your perception of fun.
But you left me with questions, that still haunt me today,
Why I can't recollect, exactly what happened that day.

The story had holes, or that's what I'm left to believe,
Such assuming barbarity, no-one could even conceive.
I can't even ask now, as our paths don't cross,
But part of my dignity still feels a loss.

I will continue to pray, for truth to prevail from a lie,
That if injustice it is, you all recollect 'till you die.
If you took something, that wasn't rightfully yours,
May they open to you, Hell's burning doors.

No More

I roll 'til I can't roll no more,
I smoke, 'til I can't smoke no more,
I drink 'til I can't drink no more,
Inside my head, a never ending war.

What's the price I've got to pay, to find some peace?
What do I have to do, for them to help me?
I've tried everything, but still, they can't see me.

Only when it becomes scandal, are they quick to point,
"Yes, she was the girl with the burnt out joint".
The soothing affects though, don't numb the pain,
I only look back now, to think that I was insane.

*The itch of sin,
the echo of desire.
The one that will lead
to the perpetual fire.*

Nothing To See?

I've become something I didn't want to be,
You turned away from something you didn't want to see.
But whilst I stayed in a world, secretly abused,
My heart couldn't point out, the one justly accused.
I tried to justify all their manipulative actions,
Whilst they removed my esteem by tremendous fractions.
I was no longer proud of the girl I'd become,
But to these daily burdens I had relentlessly succumbed.
Why had I continued, to make these excuses?
There's nothing to see here, only invisible bruises.

Rape Preach?

"You're the girl of my dreams", so where's all that gone?
Saw your eyes light up, as the moon above shone.
I knew it was lust, from the first time I heard those words,
But now there's nothing, but silence, except for the birds.

As you pulled me near, and grasped me tight,
You said, "there's no need to fear and no need to fight".
But from the first day I met you, my heart skipped a beat,
Another action, I don't wish to repeat.
'Cos adrenaline rushed, but there was no peace,
And when you weren't around, the adrenaline ceased.
From the pit of my stomach, I felt the emotion,
Your words tried to brainwash, through effective corrosion.
I didn't doubt you, but had self-belief,
So that in times like these, I could find relief.

Expectedly stayed, to see if you dared,
But all along, I was fully prepared.
So when you tried to beat me, I didn't try to escape,
In what would eventually, result in a rape.
Let you have your three blows, to see if you repent,
But my granted wishes, you so happily spent.
I gave you a chance, to feel like a man,
But to your motives, I had an ulterior plan.
Before the fourth strike, I pulled out my knife,
And without second thought, I stabbed, and I sliced.
I wanted you happy, so slashed cheek to cheek,
Now my violent storm, has reached its peak.
"Say something!" But now your screams have been silenced,
From what I call an excusable violence.
You were never a man, and that's what we've seen,
They tried to arrest me, but I got away clean.
I might have known that you would try an offence,
So I told the truth, and pleaded self-defence.

(Man's response)
"You're my property girl, da loan's through,
We married, I vowed to own you.
Da moments you make me raise my hand,
A God right to, if you don't act right too.
I take what is mine,
Da times you forget who you are.
Da times you make a contract breach,
It's not your place to try to rape preach.
You're a woman, I'm da man, so I'll teach."

(Lady's Final Word)
It's not a rape preach, it's a planned ambition,
Take a minute to hear my final decision.
You can't teach me something, that's not worth learning,
And when I'm gone, it will be you that is yearning.
The contract, was for richer and poorer, you'll love me until the
    end,
But these regulations you tried to bend.
Why? Am I lying? You broke them, the way you broke me,
After fractures, and miscarriages, I just had to flee.
I can't forgive and I can't forget,
I will kill you one day, I made that bet.
If I didn't do it, I'd become your slave,
I wasn't scared, I swore on my own grave.

(Years gone by ...)
You open the door, and I look straight at your face,
See the girl behind you, that's now taken my place.
With my eyebrows raised, I whip out my hatchet,
I've taken a slice, before you try to snatch it.
This one's so no more dead babies, can be created by you,
 This one's so you can longer screw.
Beg for mercy, on your bloody knees,
You're in debt to me, so now pay your fees.
I don't want to finish you off, that will eventually come,
But as for me, my work here, is done.
I'll let you drown, in your own blood,
The girl rushes to you and tries to stop the flood.
Suffering is the best way for you to die .....
As I walk away, oh yeah, "Good-bye!".

You Let Me Walk Away

As I walked away in the pouring rain,
You looked away and ignored my pain.
Too much hassle for you to handle,
But it was all cool when there were candles,
And music and atmosphere, in my room,
That's what you like I assume.
That was all you ever wanted,
But showed me sweetness and just fronted,
Like you would be there for ever more,
But I wasn't entirely sure with the score.
What you meant was you come when you want, and do as you please,
Use and abuse me like your fucking tease.
And then you would disappear without a trace,
And next time again you will be up in my face,
Saying you had a few problems,
And needed time, so that you could resolve them.
Do you really think that I'm brain dead?
And it's not just the fact that you wanted me in bed.

Genocide In Gaza At Christmas (Again...)

Christmas, birth of a child and world-wide peace
But innocents are still killed in rubble;
When will the loving start and hatred cease?
Just carry on living in your bubble.
War crimes and civilians' blood being shed
We all bleed the same colour – and that's red.

I can only pray that "the end is nigh"
But God is love and love's greater than hate:
For the innocents whose mouths are left dry
Life-giving water, new life to create.
Dreams, hopes and aspirations of those left
To bring hope and healing to those bereft.

Most documented Genocide is here
Not just Biblical murder by Herod;
The air is just stagnant with death and fear,
Cannot be washed away like Noah's Flood.
Can we stop the tyrants once and for all –
Not buried by bricks of a wailing wall?

5/12/24
By Saida Chowdhury & Ian Henery

4. Searching & Hopeful

Dreamers are we that manifest visions,
That only the brave think are possible.
Dreamers are we that dream visions,
That only the brave can manifest.

A Billion Stars

A billion stars and a billion tears,
I've hidden this pain for so many years.
I look upon a sombre night,
Which star will answer to my plight?

A billion years of evolution,
But nothing serves me with a solution.
I look deep, and search further inside,
As the beaming moon, soon becomes my guide.

Such beauty hanging in the navy sky,
Was it coincidence, or is that just a lie?
I call the Creator, "Please give me peace!"
"When will all this heartache cease?"
I start to tremble and then feel calm,
They say, "Our future's written in our palms".

A billion stars and a billion fears,
Now comes to a halt, my never-ending tears.

Can We?

Can we fly into oblivion, just you and me?
Can we fly to a place, where we can finally be free?
Can we fly to a space, where we don't age with time?
Can we fly to a place, where everything is fine?

Can we wander upon a garden, full of flowers and peace?
Can we wander upon a forest, where our troubles cease?
Can we wander through a waterfall, and get joyfully wet?
Can we wander to a place, that we will, never forget?

Can we drive through the wilderness, of evergreen?
Can we drive through the deserts and the magic unseen?
Can we drive through the city, with lights so bright?
Can we drive through life, with you holding me tight?

Can we swim through lagoons of turquoise clear?
Can we swim through our troubles, without shedding a tear?
Can we swim through oceans, as deep as my love?
Can we swim in the heavens, that lie above?

Defiance Exhausts Me

Defiance exhausts me …I'm standing in shame.
There's nothing I've learned and nothing I've gained.
The thrill was though, in seeking defiance …
But who had known, I had taken Satan's alliance?

He penetrated my mind, so my judgement was lacking,
And although my intentions were good, my actions were slacking.
Slowly, slowly I got strangely diverted,
From a path so straight, only blindness would conceal it.

But for my loss, The Lord has Mercy,
I was just lost; no-one had cursed me.
I begged for forgiveness and proceeded forth,
On a path seeking peace, is what I sought.

In His Infinite Wisdom, he forgave my deeds,
A lifetime of praying, on my spectacular beads.

Don't Suffer In Silence

Don't suffer in silence, when I am near,
Don't suffer in silence, there's nothing to fear.

Don't suffer in silence, when darkness looms,
Don't suffer in silence, let happiness resume.

Don't suffer in silence, I'm here my love,
Don't suffer in silence, when Heaven's above.

In The Midst Of A Dream (Grenfell x)

In the midst of dream, …I am gently woken,
"Our time has come," are the soft words spoken.
A moment of dread, makes my heart beat a flutter,
Now my worldly possessions, seem nothing but clutter.

In the midst of a dream, …I am gently shaken,
"We will be next! Fifth floor has been taken!"
A spontaneous frown rivals a gasp,
My things no longer matter, to my family I clasp.

In the midst of a dream, …I am abruptly woken,
"Our time has come!", Are shrilled, not spoken.
I jump to my feet, in a moment of hope,
I check the room for exits, but there's just too much smoke.

In the midst of a dream, I am forcefully shaken,
"We will be next! Our lives are His for the taking!"
I remember The Almighty, as I clamber to my feet,
With pious hearts wide open, I think of those we shall meet.

In the midst of a dream, I am gently woken,
"Your time is here", pure, soft words spoken.
And as I rise from my chaise of luxurious gold,
They say my story is one, that will forever be told.

Keep On Smiling

I smile because, otherwise the tears would roll down.
I smile because, otherwise there would only be a frown.
I smile because, the pain is slowly killing me.
I smile because, it's something, you just can't see.

I smile because, the people have no inkling of a clue.
I smile because, there's nothing else, I actually can do.
I smile because, it's just a matter of pride.
I smile because, I'm broken, and that's what I hide.

I smile because, the rain obscures their vision.
I smile because, it blurs my tears, in a sweet collision.
I smile because, the wind, refreshes my mind.
I smile because, it's just a way, for me to be kind.

I smile because, it's a massive part of me.
I smile because, that's my fractured reality.
I smile because, the children, learn from what they see.
I smile because, it gives stress, it's invisibility.

I smile because, there's no-one, out there to help me.
I smile because, I have faith, in The One Almighty.
I smile because I know, patience is the key.
I smile because, one day, I know I'll be free.

My Refuge

My subterranean refuge, is a space in time,
Grotesquely beautiful and uniquely sublime.

The doors remain closed, when life is bliss,
They allow my entry, if chance takes a miss.

This dwelling is temporary, but awaits my arrival,
It's an essential retreat, for my mental survival.

Once I reside there, there's no limit to my stay,
And every moment avoids, a monotonous day.

There's no windows or crevices, to let light in,
But that's what I prefer there, atmospherically dim.

That's what I yearn, when my soul needs a break,
It becomes my refuge, for my mental state.

The comfort is knowing, it's a space for one,
It's an abode away from home, to which I always can run.

But the residence here, is not a permanent stay,
It's designed to temporarily, leave struggles at bay.

I enjoy my refuge, when it welcomes me,
A place to seek solace and find clarity.

My subterranean refuge is a space in time,
Grotesquely beautiful and uniquely sublime.

I Don't See The Scars

I wish you could see yourself through my eyes ...
I don't see the scars ...
I see paths that led to escape; avenues that led to freedom,
And routes that led you to become,
The beautiful person you are today.

I don't see the scars ...
I see a myriad of beautiful contours, vestiges of endless
 adventures,
Traces of overcome battles ...
Remnants of a past, longed to be forgotten.

I don't see the scars ...
I see symbols of overwhelming bravery, remains of undeniable
 resilience,
Beautiful waves that glisten,
Reminders of a new life.

I wish you could see yourself through my eyes ...
I wish your scars didn't return you to a time,
When your only consolation was to hold yourself in the darkness.
I wish they didn't ... for I am here now, beside you.

Your scars are not to me, what they are to you.
They are not the ugly memories of a troubled past.
They are but residues of untold stories.
I am here ... and your scars are not ugly to me, as they are to
 you ...
Kintsugi on a human form ...
I wish you could just see yourself, through my eyes.

Plan Of Action

There was a plan of action, which I didn't take,
I resolved to smile, even though it was fake.
Whilst my world crumbled inside its walls,
There wasn't a soul, that answered my calls.

But they are quick to judge with their fingers,
All full of advice, but nothing necessary lingers.
I'm full of shame but also committed,
To regain myself from a past omitted.

I have walked on shells, but my feet are hardened,
And though I still feel pain, your sins are pardoned.
I can't shake the thought, even though I fear it,
I tried the slipper, but it just didn't fit.

I'll rebuild my world, from the remaining fragments,
My soul needs relighting from too long being stagnant.
I've got my armour and shield at the ready,
And though I'm shaking inside, my posture is steady.

With my faith in The One,
I resolve to be true.
There's nothing but prayers and best wishes for you.

The Worth of Women

International Women's Day Panel – University of Wolverhampton

I stood in the shadows and watched them talk,
How for centuries for recognition we earnestly fought.
But these glass ceilings conceal nothing,
We still saw the sky. For without self-belief,
There's no way, to just fly.

They put barriers in our way,
To dissuade us from trying,
But we wouldn't give up,
Even through all the tears we've been crying.

We struggled with the powers,
But defied their expectations.
We weren't put here to blindly follow,
Archaic regulations.

Resilience is what we had,
In order to prove to the world.
That monumental footsteps had been taken,
From progress of becoming a great woman from a girl.

We don't deny our struggles,
We are here to inspire.
From continual promotion of ambition,
We will never retire.

We've defied their barriers,
We've reached new heights.
We didn't get to where we've gotten,
Without endless sleepless nights.

So don't discount our value,
We're paving the way.
For new generations to recognise,
The worth of women every day.

Find strength in the storm
There's blessing in the rain,
Everything is temporary
Even your pain.

About Saida Chowdhury

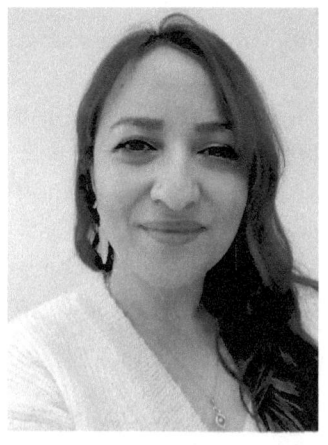

Saida, who graduated from Queen Mary, University of London, has been writing poetry for over 20 years. Her debut collection, *Broken Minds*, will be accompanied with poetry workshops across Birmingham on the theme of mental health and the aim of removing the stigma.

Saida was born in Bangladesh and came to the UK as a baby before growing up in West London. She moved to Birmingham over 18 years ago after getting married and is the mother of 2 teenage boys.

The first time that she had performed spoken word in front of an audience only took place on November 27th, 2024, for Words of Wisdom at Café Royale in Wolverhampton. Since then, she has had the confidence to read more of her work for the Human Rights Celebration Day on 10th December at the University of Wolverhampton, The RICNIC New Year Arts Festival, The Ian Henery Show Black Country Xtra, The Verve Open Mic, The Delves Baptist Church charity fundraiser, Katie Fitzgerald's, West Midlands House - Netwalking, Robertos, Poetry Breakfast and The International Women's Day Celebration at the University of Wolverhampton alongside Sureena Brackenridge MP for Wolverhampton North East who has written the foreword for *Broken Minds*. Saida was part of the Poets Against Racism Collective at the first publishing fair held by Staffordshire Poet Laureate, Scarlett Ward. Her latest feature was being asked to be the poet for Legacy West Midlands at their 'Pohela Boishak' event which is a traditional Bangladeshi festival welcoming in the spring and New Year. For this event Saida wrote and performed her first ever poem in Bengali.

Her debut poetry book, *Broken Minds* explores various themes of love, depression, loss and faith, but they are all entwined and understood by her personal understanding of the Japanese art form of *kintsugi*.

"We are all broken," explains Saida, "and there is a Japanese word, *kintsugi* which means 'Golden Joinery'. It`s a traditional Japanese art of mending broken pottery and ceramics using either precious metal liquids or lacquer with gold dusting. *Kintsugi* beautifies the breakage and treats it as an inspirational part of the object's history and the broken pot not as something to discard but as something more precious than it was before".

Saida's intention is to apply this philosophy to human trauma and scars both physical, mental and emotional.

Her message to people is "Your scars are not ugly, they are beautiful parts of you and your history that need to be embraced in order to heal, help and grow.

She began using poetry over twenty years ago after witnessing the injustices of the aftermath of 9/11 and trying to understand the root causes of the injustices that exist in the world.

www.ingramcontent.com/pod-product-compliance
Lightning Source LLC
Chambersburg PA
CBHW022213090526
44584CB00013BA/849